Copyright Page

Cover Designed by Jessica Dumas.

This Book is Dedicated to Ruth M. Morris

April 3, 1921 to September 12, 2017

This book is being dedicated to my grandmother who was a believer in home remedies and inspired me to write this book. She was a loving and caring person who was devout in her faith. I miss our long conversations sitting on her porch while visiting her southern home in a small town in Georgia. She would tell me of home remedies that she used whenever I told her of any health issues or pain I was experiencing.

My grandmother had a big garden in her backyard. I remember many times she would send me to pick catnip or other plants for certain illnesses or health complaints. She would boil them for tea or other home remedies. This book includes home remedies that she used for many of her own health problems along with others I have collected.

I have used many of her home remedies successfully and have passed them on to friends and family, which makes me want to share them with everyone because of the large amount of success stories I have received. It is my firm belief that home remedies are very useful and I sincerely hope that some of these will be beneficial to you and your family.

I also wish to thank my mother for her continuous support.

Please feel free to leave a review of this book with the publisher. For more healthy tips please follow my blog at https://www.rosarm4u.com

May your life be enriched by using these home remedies.

Rosalind Armstrong

Medical Disclaimer

This book is not intended as a substitute for the medical advice of physicians. The reader should regularly consult a physician in matters relating to his/her health and particularly with respect to any symptoms that may require diagnosis or medical attention.

The contents of this book are for informational purposes only. You should always consult with your physician or other qualified health provider before using any home remedy in this book or if you have any questions regarding using these remedies for your individual medical condition.

Many people have used these remedies for years but that does not mean that you could not have an allergy to something in a remedy. It is important that you understand that any essential oils can be potent and should be kept away from your eyes and away from children. Just because they are an oil does not mean you can cook with them.

The author of this book will not be held responsible for the results of any remedies you try and will not be responsible for any medical costs incurred from using these remedies. Reliance on any home remedy in this book is solely at the reader's risk.

If you have any distressing reaction to any of the home remedies in this book, call 911 immediately.

Table of Contents

Chapter 1: About Home Remedies

History

Home remedies can be traced back in history to ancestors of several cultures for thousands of years. Home remedies use plants, herbs, roots, fruits and vegetables as an alternative to medication to help alleviate common health problems. About 30% of drugs today are still being synthesized from plants.

The ancient Egyptians used honey as a remedy for high blood pressure, cramps and earache. Long before the expression 'an apple a day keeps the doctor away' became popular, apple cider vinegar was used to treat several ailments and was even believed to be the fountain of youth. It was also used as a disinfectant and antiseptic.

One of the first home remedies discovered by the Chinese was how therapeutic ginger is for nausea, inflammation, and to improve the immune system. Orientals also used celery to treat high blood pressure, which science has proved relaxes the muscle linings of blood vessels.

One of the most useful remedies started during World War I when garlic was pounded into water and then applied to wounds on a bed of moss for dressing.

The fact that several home remedies have been used for centuries shows how safe they are as a form of first-line treatment, but they are not intended to replace the treatments from a physician.

Home Remedies vs. Modern Medicine

There has been a debate for several years on modern medicine versus home remedies. Just like my grandmother, millions of people are using home remedies for several different conditions. Why is this? There are several reasons, but the biggest reason is due to how modern medical practices are causing persons to turn to using home remedies for many common problems that are not emergencies or related to severe diseases. To point this out, some of the reasons are as follows:

Side Effects of Medicine

Medicines of today are mostly made of synthetic chemicals that can have negative side effects for many people. Some of these side effects can be dangerous to the point of causing death.

High Costs of Medicine

Most medicine today come with huge price tags that many people cannot afford especially in developing nations. If a person has insurance, it helps pay the cost but even then, many insurance companies do not cover the full cost and the co-pay can be hundreds or even thousands of dollars. In addition, insurance has become so expensive that millions cannot afford it and they go either without food to pay for medication or just do not get the medication. Either choice can be dangerous.

Lack of Preventive Health in Modern Medicine

Modern medical personnel normally emphasize the cure rather than prevention. Medicine has become a multi-billion-dollar market and profits seem to be more important than helping people be healthy. Insurance companies are getting better about covering preventative check-ups.

If insurance does not cover it, this doesn't mean that you should not have a preventive health or physical check-up every year with a physician. The yearly check-up is important for screening cancers and having blood tests that can show disease such as diabetes or heart disease.

Benefits of Home Remedies

Due to how many people feel about modern medicine, many have concluded that home remedies are like a stepping stone to modern medicine. In other words, home remedies can be used before seeking medical help. Many people suffer from minor ailments such as headaches, minor back or joint pain, skin issues, flu or allergies that can be benefited by home remedies.

Without the centuries of use of home remedies, medicine would not have advanced to the degree they have. The only thing about home remedies that may not be appreciated is that they take longer to work than modern medicine. Some of the benefits are as follows:

Low Side Effects

When you can take something for a back ache, the flu, an allergy, sunburn or any other minor health problem, you don't have to worry about side effects if it's something you normally eat from your kitchen.

Less Doctor Visits

Some people think that just because you use home remedies, you don't need to go to the doctor, but this is not true. Most home remedies are used first before going to the doctor. This works only with conditions that are not emergencies or considered serious.

There are some doctors who commend their patients for trying home remedies first as it could diminish or even stop symptoms. If you don't need to go to the doctor's office, just think of the hassle you have avoided dealing with waiting, paying, or maybe even rude office staff. However, if your symptoms get worse after trying home remedies, you must seek medical attention.

Inexpensive

Home remedy ingredients are normally lower priced than medications even when buying organic. With less doctor visits, your out-of-pocket costs will be lower, and you may not have to go to the pharmacy and pay a co-pay for a drug.

Home Remedies vs. Alternatives

It is important to explain that home remedies are not the same as other alternative ways of medicine such as herbal therapy, homeopathic, or holistic remedies. Many times, they are mixed up or mistaken for each other because alternatives use many home or natural remedies. The word 'natural' is used so much in the food industry that it's confusing. Below are some short explanations of each alternative so that you will not mix them up with home remedies.

Herbal (or Herbal Therapy, Herbalism)

Herbal products are made from plants, plant roots or leaves. They are free from chemicals but not necessarily free from pesticides. Herbalism is the study of botany and the use of plants intended for medicinal purposes or for supplementing a diet. Vitamins and supplements contain herbal products, some of which are recommended by medical physicians and covered by insurance.

Homeopathic

Homeopathic remedies use plants, minerals, and animal products whereas home remedies are usually only plant based. Neither are not necessarily free from pesticides unless certified organic. Homeopathic remedies are products that are vigorously shaken with water to allow dilution that is absorbed better. It is believed that the body will cure itself if these products are used to stimulate the healing process.

Holistic

Holistic remedies are usually given by a holistic doctor who believes all parts of a person's body need to be in balance including physical, emotional, or spiritual. It includes a combination of several therapies such as acupuncture, chiropractic, massage, spiritual counseling, and western medications.

Warnings

You need to be aware that homeopathic and holistic alternatives advertise that they sell home or natural remedies, so it can be confusing. There are many websites that sell products labeled home or natural remedies that make a massive profit from them. Beware that they are processed products and are not the type of remedies that are in this book.

Home vs. Natural Remedies

Home remedies are called 'home' due to the ingredients being found normally in the home or naturally grown in a garden and used by the immediate family in that home. The only other remedy names that should be used in place of the word 'home' in this book are in-home, homemade, or natural remedies. They are normally grown without chemicals or pesticides.

Beware that natural and organic are not necessarily the same. Natural foods may be grown with pesticides and not certified organic. If you want to be sure they are free of pesticides, always make sure they are certified organic.

Where to Buy Home Remedy Ingredients

For those of us that are not able to grow our own garden, home remedy ingredients can be found at a local farmer's market, health food stores, supermarket, or specialty grocery stores that specialize in natural and organic foods such as Trader Joes or Whole Foods Market.

Recommendations

To be 100 percent sure home remedy plants are organic, you can grow many herbs and vegetables in your own garden. If you want to start an organic garden, there are several online websites you can go to for help.

It is recommended that when trying out one remedy that you do not immediately try another one if that doesn't work. Wait until the next day to try another. I included a variety of remedies because everyone has different reactions so some of these may not do anything for you but don't give up. Try a different remedy with different ingredients.

Because you don't know which one is going to work for you, it's a good idea to make a note once you try a remedy as to if it helps or not. Having a book like this is helpful because you can keep track of the ones you try, whereas if you get one off the internet, you may not remember where it came from.

Helpful Aids

This book includes a glossary in Chapter 9 explaining many of the ingredients used in the home remedies included to help those who do not understand what they are and what they can be used for. If there are any terms not listed in the glossary, you can search for them on the internet.

At the end of the book in Chapter 10 is an index of home remedy ingredients to make it easy for you to find certain remedies that the ingredients are used in.

This book contains 120 solutions to 75 health issues, which may sound like a vast amount but there are many, many more as you can see by just doing simple searches on the internet. The ones included in this book are ones chosen to be most effective for common health issues.

May you find something that will relieve some of your pain and suffering or other health issues you may have.

Chapter 2: Remedies for Pain/Inflammation

Many painful and inflamed conditions can be reduced with home remedies unless the problem is severe enough for treatment by a specialist or medical facility.

Back pain is one of the major causes of missed work and visits to the doctor or hospital. Whether it is a herniated disc or sciatica, the pain can cause your daily activities and sleep to be disrupted. If it is severe enough, it is the third most common reason for back surgery.

Many back problems such as pain and inflammation come on slowly due to several possible factors such as carrying or lifting a lot, standing, or sitting all day. Acute back pain can strike from lifting heavy objects improperly, bending or stretching too far, falling or other injuries.

When the pain is acute, it has been proven that applying ice packs for 20 minutes every 40 minutes for the first day works well for bringing down the inflammation. After that heat can be applied but not for more than 20 minutes at a time or inflammation can return. If this and the home remedies do not relieve most of the pain in 2-4 days, going to your physician is recommended.

Arthritis affects over 50 million people and is the most common reason for disability. One common complaint is gout, which is a type of arthritis that targets the joints. Bursitis and tendinitis are other reason for joint pain that is usually the result of overuse, injury, age or repetitive motions. Fibromyalgia and many auto-immune diseases such as Lupus and Multiple Sclerosis also have joint pain that can be debilitating.

Below are several home remedies that can be used to relieve the pain and inflammation due to different types of arthritis, bursitis, tendinitis, sprains and strains, as well as fibromyalgia. Also, there are specific remedies for pain/inflammation in different parts of the body, such as back, neck, legs, feet, and joint pain.

Hot/Cold Drink Recipes for Pain/Inflammation

1) Ginger Tea

Ingredients:

1 tsp turmeric powder

2 Tbsp ginger, grated

1 C water

2 tsp raw honey

Directions:

Boil the water, add turmeric and ginger, steep for 7-9 minutes. Strain and add honey. Stir until dissolved completely and drink while warm.

2) Apple Cider Vinegar Tea

Ingredients:

2 tsp apple cider vinegar (unfiltered)

2 tsp honey

1 cup water

Sprinkle of cinnamon

Directions:

Heat water to boiling, add apple cider vinegar and honey, stir until dissolved. Cool until able to drink warm. Sprinkle with cinnamon if desired. Repeat twice a day.

3) Grape Juice for Arthritis

Ingredients:

1 Tbsp of liquid pectin (or apple cider vinegar unfiltered)

8 oz. 100% grape juice

Directions:

Mix and drink 1-2 times daily. Give it a week or two for results.

4) Turmeric Milk for Pain

Ingredients:

1 cup milk warmed

1 tsp ground turmeric

½ tsp ground ginger

Directions:

Warm milk in microwave to drinking temperature and add turmeric and ginger until dissolved. Drink 3 times a day.

5) Raw Potato Juice for Arthritis

Ingredients:

1 potato, peeled and chopped

Directions:

Using a food processor or by hand, mash potato and press out one or two teaspoons of the juice. Take before eating meals. Do not store extra for more than a few hours. Best when fresh. The juice of raw potato is regarded as an excellent remedy for inflammation from arthritis.

6) Lemony Turmeric Tea

Ingredients

1 cup water

¼ tsp turmeric powder

¼ tsp ground cinnamon

¼ tsp ground ginger

½ tsp raw honey

1 Tbsp lemon juice

Directions

Heat water in microwave or pan until almost boiling. Add the spices, honey, lemon juice, and stir to dissolve. Remove and cover with a lid. Let sit for 10 minutes. Stir and drink when cool. Drink once or twice daily.

7) White Willow Tea

Ingredients:

2 tsp of powdered white willow bark

1 cup of water

Honey or lemon to taste

Directions:

Bring water to a boil, reduce to a simmer and add white willow bark. Let it infuse for 10-15 minutes, remove from heat and steep for 30 minutes. Add honey and/or lemon and drink twice daily.

8) Very Pink Smoothie

Ingredients

1 cup strawberries (fresh or frozen)

½ cup beets, peeled and chopped

1 cup 100% cranberry juice

½ in. of ginger root, peeled (or 1 tsp powder)

1 Tbsp honey

½ tsp cinnamon

Ice (optional)

Directions

Add all ingredients to blender, pulse until smooth. Have once daily.

9) Pineapple Honey Drink

Ingredients

2 slices fresh pineapple (or ¼ cup frozen pieces)

2 cups water

½ tsp raw honey

1 tsp turmeric

Directions

Place all ingredients in a blender and blend until smooth. Drink 2-3 times a day.

---

10) Nettle Leaf & Turmeric Tea

Ingredients:

1 cup water

1 Tbsp nettle leaf dried

1 tsp turmeric

Directions:

Heat water to boiling, add nettle leaf and turmeric, steep for 5 minutes. Strain into another cup using fine mesh strainer. Drink up to 4 times a day for relief.

---

11) Alfalfa Tea

Ingredients:

1 cup water

1 tsp alfalfa leaves

2 tsp lemon juice

1 tsp honey

Directions:

Heat water to almost boiling, add lemon juice and honey, steep for 10-15 minutes. Drink once a day two days a week. Too much may cause bloating. Ask your doctor before using alfalfa if you have diabetes or any auto-immune disease.

---

12) Dandelions for Arthritis

Ingredients:

3 tsp of fresh dandelion leaves (or 1 teaspoon of dried)

1 tsp honey

1 cup of boiling water

A handful of fresh leaves (if making a salad)

A dash of extra virgin olive oil (if making a salad)

Directions:

Heat water and add dandelion leaves, steep for 10 minutes. Strain, add honey and drink twice daily. For making a salad, toss the greens in with another recipe or gently sautéed to soften up a bit.

Rubs & Tubs for Pain/Inflammation

13) Warm Cayenne Rub

Ingredients:

1 Pint apple cider vinegar (unfiltered)

1 tsp cayenne pepper

Directions:

Boil apple cider vinegar, add cayenne pepper, cool. Using cloth while wearing rubber gloves, carefully apply to affected area. Cayenne pepper can cause skin irritation so if it feels like it's burning, stop immediately. (see glossary warning)

14) Potato Rub

Ingredients:

3 medium potatoes (or more depending on the size of area you wish to treat)

Directions:

Boil potatoes in their skins until tender. Place them in some muslin and mash. Apply the warm sack to the painful area. Remove once it has cooled down completely.

15) Almond Oil Rub

Ingredients:

2 Tbsp almond oil

1 tsp cayenne pepper

Directions:

Mix in a small bowl and apply to affected area using gloves. Leave on for 10 minutes. Wash off with soap and warm water. Repeat up to three times a day until pain subsides. (see glossary warning)

16) Lavender Oil Rub for Neck Pain

Ingredients:

4 ice cubes

5 drops lavender oil

Directions:

Place ice cubs in small towel and hold against painful area for 10 minutes. Massage lavender oil into area. Repeat every 2-3 hours until pain subsides.

17) Backache Tub Soak

Ingredients:

1 cup Epsom salts

1 tsp cayenne pepper

Directions:

Add Epsom salt and pepper to warm bathwater to soak for 30 minutes. Repeat twice a day. Be careful not to get into eyes. (see glossary warning on cayenne pepper)

Eating Your Way Away from Pain/Inflammation

There are several foods that are good for relief of arthritis. It's a proven fact that foods high in omega-3 fatty acids help reduce inflammation. Eating lots of fruits and vegetables can help prevent rheumatoid arthritis. Some of the top foods for the pain and inflammation of arthritis are: fatty fish such as salmon, garlic, broccoli, ginger, turmeric, walnuts, spinach, berries, olive oil, grapes, beets, cherries or tart cherry juice. Research has shown that the Mediterranean diet, which uses a lot of olive oil can lower inflammation, so I've included a Mediterranean salad below.

18) Mediterranean Salad

Ingredients:

Dressing

3 Tbsp fresh lemon juice

1 Tbsp apple cider vinegar

3 Tbsp extra virgin olive oil

1/4 tsp dried mustard

1/2 tsp garlic powder

1/8 tsp cayenne pepper

Salt to taste

Salad

1 6 oz. can albacore tuna (or 6 oz. salmon)

1 cucumber, peeled and chopped

1 large tomato, chopped

1/2 cup fresh broccoli spears

1/4 cup fresh red onion, finely chopped

1/2 cup purple or black grapes, sliced in half

1/2 red bell pepper, chopped

2 cups fresh spinach

1 cup romaine or other lettuce, chopped

1/2 red cabbage, finely sliced

1/2 cup chopped walnuts

Directions:

In a medium bowl, combine salad dressing ingredients and whisk together thoroughly and. (see glossary warning on cayenne)

In large bowl, mix all salad ingredients except walnuts, cover, and refrigerate for at least chill 30 minutes. Toss with dressing and top with walnuts before serving.

---

19) Eggplant Mash

Ingredients:

1 medium eggplant

Extra virgin olive oil spray

1 glove garlic, minced

2 Tbsp castor oil (or olive oil)

1 tsp turmeric

½ tsp cumin (or cayenne pepper)

½ tsp coriander

Sea salt to taste

Directions:
Cut eggplant into bite size chunks, spray with olive oil, bake at 375 degrees for 25-30 minutes until softened. Mash and fry with garlic in oil adding spices as it's frying until browned. Serve plain or on a bed of spinach. Eat once a day for two to three months for relief.

20) Curried Chicken & Cherry Salad

Ingredients (for 4):
3 Tbsp light mayonnaise
1 Tbsp apple cider vinegar (unfiltered)
1-1/2 tsp curry powder
1 tsp ginger (fresh or powder)
1/2 tsp turmeric
2 cups cooked chicken, cubed
1 cup fresh cherries, pitted and sliced
1 medium avocado, peeled, pitted and diced
1/4 small red onion, diced
2 Tbsp cilantro, minced
Salt & pepper to taste
1/2 cup walnuts, chopped fine
Handful of spinach or lettuce leaves

Directions:
Mix the mayonnaise, apple cider vinegar, curry powder, ginger and turmeric in large bowl. Fold in the chicken, cherries, avocado, onion and cilantro. Add more mayo if needed. Season to taste with salt and pepper. Sprinkle with the walnuts and serve on a bed of spinach or lettuce leaves.

21) Autumn Beet Salad

Serves: 2

Ingredients:
2 cups beets (about 2 large beets), roasted
4 cups spring mix salad greens
1/2 cup organic walnuts, chopped

2 Tbsp pomegranate seeds (or raspberries)
1/2 cup extra virgin olive oil
1/4 cup apple cider vinegar
Sea salt and lemon pepper to taste

Directions:
Preheat oven to 450 degrees. Rinse beets and trim the beet greens
close to the beet. Dry and put on baking sheet lined with foil and
cover with foil. Roast for 45 minutes to an hour, or until tender.
Allow to cool to the touch and peel the skin. Slice the beets thinly
and set aside to cool to room temperature. Top the salad greens
with chopped raw walnuts, pomegranate seeds, and the beet slices.
In a small jar, shake the olive oil and vinegar, drizzle over the
salads and season to taste.

22) Apple Cider Vinaigrette

Ingredients:
1/4 cup apple cider vinegar
3 tablespoons extra virgin olive oil
1 clove minced garlic
1 tablespoon honey or maple syrup
1 teaspoon Dijon mustard
Sea salt & pepper to taste

Directions:
Place all ingredients into a salad dressing jar with lid. Shake until
well combined. Cool in the refrigerator until ready to use. For an
oil-free dressing, use orange juice instead of oil.

Home Remedies for Sciatica

Sciatica is a combination of symptoms caused by pressure being put
on the sciatic nerve and runs from the lower back down through
the buttocks and the back of the leg. It is can be an excruciating pain
and is brought on for different reasons such as injury or strain of
the low back, pelvis or hip causing inflammation of the nerve.

Besides trying the following remedies and those for back pain above, there are stretches that will help prevent and reduce sciatica (https://gethealthyu.com/stretches-to-relieve-sciatica-pain). If it is severe enough, you may need medication to relax the sciatic nerve and a physician should be consulted.

23) Ivy Rub

Ingredients:

2 handfuls of ivy leaf, chopped

2 handfuls of bran

1 cup water

Directions:

Mix the ivy and bran into water stirring to make a paste. Warm over low heat for 10 minutes. Apply to low back area with a cloth and leave for 30 minutes.

24) Sciatic Soak

Ingredients:

1 cup Epsom salts

1 tsp cayenne pepper

Directions:

Add Epsom salt and pepper to warm bathwater to soak for 30 minutes. Repeat twice a day. Be careful not to get cayenne pepper in eyes (see glossary warning).

Home Remedies for Lower Extremities

25) Almond Lavender Rub for Leg Pain

Ingredients:

5 drops lavender oil

2 Tbsp almond oil

Directions:

Mix together and massage into legs for 5 minutes and then wash them clean with warm water. Repeat daily to treat restless leg syndrome or leg pain. It will also help to soak in the bathtub with some Epsom salt after this treatment.

26) Hot/Cold Soak for Aching Feet

Ingredients:
1/2 cup Epsom salts
1/2 cup apple cider vinegar (unfiltered)
Peppermint or eucalyptus oil

Directions:
Fill two foot basins – 1 with hot water and 1 with ice water. Put half of the Epsom salt and vinegar in each of the basins. Place feet in the basin with the hot water and soak for 5 minutes. Remove and soak it in the cold water for 5 minutes. Do this repeatedly until you feel relief. Soaking your feet alternately in hot and cold water will cause the blood vessels in the feet to dilate and constrict. This jump starts circulation of blood in the feet thereby giving the feet relief. After soaking, rub feet with peppermint or eucalyptus oil. Put socks on and keep feet elevated for a couple hours. Staying off your feet for a while will also help.

27) Boswellia Smoothie for Knee Joint Pain/Popping

Ingredients:
1 cup organic coconut or almond milk
1/2 to 1 cup frozen organic blueberries or cherries
2 Tbsp freshly ground flaxseed
1 Tbsp Boswellia serrata powder (or 2 tsp oil)
2 tsp turmeric
2 tsp cinnamon
1/4 tsp probiotic powder
Chopped ice (optional)

Directions:
Place all ingredients in a blender. Blend for one minute until smooth. If smoothie is too thick, thin with purified water or coconut milk. Serve immediately – makes 1 serving.

28) Papaya for Corns

Ingredients:

4-5 drops of peppermint oil

1/2 tsp papaya juice

1 slice of lemon

Directions:

Add peppermint oil to footbath of warm water and soak for 30 minutes. Dry well and apply papaya juice over the corn and cover with bandage. At night place lemon slice on corn and wrap with gauze. Remove in the morning and repeat the soak and papaya rub 3 times a day until corn disappears.

29) Home Remedies for Athlete's Foot

Rub tea tree oil between toes. Put crushed garlic glove into dry socks before bed. Raw garlic is known to kill foot fungus. Grapefruit seed extract is reported to have anti-fungal effects. Add drops of grapefruit seed extract to wet hands and apply it to the feet two to three times per day. The cheapest and most effective treatment is bicarbonate of soda. Sprinkle a little between your toes before you put on socks and shoes.

30) Gingko Biloba and Aloe Vera for Edema

Ingredients:

1/2 cup coconut oil (or almond oil)

1/2 cup aloe vera gel

15 drops rosemary essential oil

20 drops gingko biloba extract

Directions:

In small bowl, add all and mix well. Cover and store in cool dry place. Massage into swollen legs starting from ankles and working up. Repeat twice a day until symptoms subside.

Chapter 3: Cold and Flu Home Remedies

It seems like as soon as the weather cools down, the colds and flu heat up the hospital ERs and doctor offices. That is usually because school is back in session and those germs are running wild as the children are running down the hallways touching everyone and everything. Not only that, once we turn on our heat, the germs are happy because they get to multiply like crazy in the warmth but with a few home remedies, you can fight them off.

Remedies for Colds/Sore Throat/Cough

31) Catnip Tea for Colds and Other Viruses

Make tea out of dried catnip leaves by boiling until water is a light brown color. Drink approximately 6 ounces to drive out colds. Can also help drive out the measles and mumps. Can be sweetened with up to 1 tablespoon of honey to desired taste.

32) Mustard Steam Inhaler

Ingredients:

1 tsp dried mustard

3 cups water

Directions:

At the first sign of a cold and fever, pour hot water into bowl. Add dried mustard to a bowl, stir to dissolve. Inhale steam being careful not to get too close. This will clear phlegm and draw any infection and congestion out of the chest.

33) Apple Cider Vinegar for Sore Throat and Colds

Ingredients:

1-2 tsp apple cider vinegar (unfiltered)

1 cup water

Directions:

Heat water to be warm, add apple cider vinegar. Drink 1-3 times a day. Also gargling with straight apple cider vinegar will help sore throat. Apple cider vinegar is a natural antibacterial.

34) Lemonade Cold Remedy

Ingredients:

This recipe makes 6 cups.

6 cups water
3 cups fresh lemon balm leaves (or 1 cup dried)
4 lemons (juiced to equal about 1 cup of juice)
3 Tbsp honey

Directions:

Heat up water to boiling. Put the lemon balm leaves in the bottom of 2-quart pitcher. Crush the leaves with plastic/wooden spoon. Pour the hot water over leaves and let it steep for 1 hour. Then strain the leaves, add the lemon juice and honey. Stir well and let it cool somewhat for tea if using for cold or headache. If you want as a cold refreshing lemonade for a fever or sore throat, refrigerate until cold and add ice. Each cup has only 36 calories.

35) Lemon Honey Tea

Ingredients:
2 lemons
1 tsp honey
1 cup water

Directions:

Squeeze juice of lemons into a mug, pour hot water into mug, add honey and stir. Cool to drinking temperature, drink 2-3 times a day.

36) Ginger Cold/Fever Remedy

Ingredients:
Foot tub of water as hot as you can stand it
2 tsp fresh ginger
(or use a few drops of ginger oil or peppermint essential oil)

Directions:
Heat water, pour into foot basin, stir in ginger. Soak feet until water cools off. This will draw congestion and fever out of head.

37) Lemon Congestion Relief

Ingredients:

¼ cup squeezed lemon juice

¼ cup apple cider vinegar (unfiltered)

½ tsp ginger powder

½ tsp cayenne pepper

3 Tbsp raw honey

Directions:

In small saucepan pour lemon juice and apple cider vinegar, bring to a boil and simmer for 2 minutes, remove from stove. Add ginger and pepper, stir to dissolve, add honey and mix well and pour into a container with a cover to store in refrigerator. Take 1 orf 2 tablespoons of mixture every day until congestion clears. Be careful not to get cayenne pepper in eyes (see glossary warning).

38) Cinnamon Sore Throat Soother

Ingredients:

1 tsp of cardamom powder

1 tsp of ground cinnamon

1 cup of hot water

Directions:

Add cardamom and cinnamon to the hot water and let it steep for 5 minutes. Strain the water into another cup using a fine mesh strainer. Drink up to 4 times a day until the sore throat subsides.

39) Cabbage Compress for Cough/Bronchitis

Ingredients:

4 cabbage leaves

1 onion

Directions:

Using a rolling pin, crush cabbage leaves until the juice starts to seep out and roast onions until soft. Place on chest area and cover with a towel. Place a warm blanket over to keep in place for 20-30 minutes every few hours until cough subsides.

40) Ginger & Honey for Bronchitis

Ingredients:

1 tsp of ground ginger

1 tsp of Manuka honey

1 cup of hot water

Directions:

Add ginger and honey to the hot water and let it steep for 5 minutes. Drink up to 4 times a day until the symptoms subside. Manuka honey is a powerful antiviral and can help to fight many of the viruses that cause bronchitis.

Home Remedies for Flu

41) Ginger & Lemon for Flu

Ingredients:

1 Tbsp ground ginger

1 Tbsp lemon juice

1 tsp manuka honey

1 cup hot water

Directions:

Bring water to boil, add ginger, lemon juice and honey. Stir and steep for 5 minutes. Drink 4 times a day until flue subsides.

42) Peppermint & Cloves for Vomiting

Ingredients:

1 Tbsp dried peppermint

1 tsp clove powder

1 cup hot water

Directions:

Bring water to boil, add peppermint and clove powder, let it steep for 5 minutes. Strain into another cup using a fine mesh strainer. Drink up to 4 times per day until the vomiting subsides.

Chapter 4: Head Pain Home Remedies

Most people have experienced headaches at some time in their life. They may be caused by tension, stress, sensitivities to light or sounds, alcohol, sinus problems or may be a sign of a cold or flu coming or hypertension. You can also get a headache for a few days if you are a coffee or cola drinker and stop drinking caffeine.

A migraine headache is more than just a serious headache. It is a neurological disorder which includes a pounding headache along with visual disturbance, nausea and vomiting. If you have a headache that continues for any length of time or that is unusually painful, see a doctor.

Home Remedies for Handling Headaches

43) Mint Coffee Yogurt Parfait for Headache

Ingredients:

3 tsp brewed coffee (dark or strong)

1 cup plain Greek yogurt

¼ cup walnuts (chopped)

¼ cup dark chocolate mints (chopped)

Garnish: Fresh Organic Chocolate Mint Leaf (optional)

Directions:

In 8-10 oz. glass, layer the yogurt, walnuts, and chocolate mints alternating until you get to the top. Garnish with fresh chocolate mint leaf.

44) Essential Oils for Sinus Headache

Ingredients:

2-3 drops pine essential oil

2-3 drops eucalyptus essential oil

1-2 drops rosemary and/or thyme essential oil

Hot water in vaporizer or bowl

1-2 drops peppermint and/or lavender essential oils

Directions:

Add the essential oils of pine, eucalyptus, rosemary or thyme, either on their own or in combination to use in vaporizer or put in a bowl and hold head over it. Make a compress out of plain water and peppermint or lavender oils. Apply compress to the forehead. Lie down and breathe in the aroma in a quiet darkened room with no distractions for at least an hour. Keep applying the compress while hot. If this doesn't help within a few days and you have a fever, consult a physician as you may have a sinus infection and need antibiotics.

45) Peppermint Oil Compress for Headache

Ingredients:

10 tsp apple cider vinegar (unfiltered)
5-6 drops peppermint essential oil
Clean piece of cloth

Directions:

Place apple cider vinegar in refrigerator to get it as cold as possible. Pour it onto clean cloth, add drops of peppermint oil and let soak for 10 minutes. Squeeze out excess fluid and place on forehead for 15-20 minutes. Return compress to refrigerator to get cold. Repeat until you get relief. Peppermint oil is one of the most effective essential oils for headache.

46) Ginger for Migraines

Ingredients:

1/8 tsp organic ground ginger or 1/4 tsp freshly grated ginger root
1 cup water

Directions:

Add ginger to the hot water and let it steep on low heat for at least 10 minutes. Drink up to 4 times a day until the symptoms subside. If you are prone to migraines, prepare tea and store in the refrigerator so as soon as you feel one coming on, heat and drink.

Ginger tea has been proven to be as effective at preventing migraines as some medications.

Other ways to use ginger to fight migraines is to make a mixture of ginger oil and almond oil to massage into temples as soon as you feel one coming on. Also, soaking your feet in fresh ginger with peppermint oil will draw the blood away from your head.

Remedies for Ear, Tooth and Eye Problems

47) Garlic for Earache

Ingredients:
1 clove garlic
1 Tbsp extra virgin olive oil
Cotton balls

Directions:
Crush the garlic and mix into olive oil that is warmed up for 15 minutes. Strain liquid into small dish. Soak a cotton ball in the liquid and place it inside the outer earlobe for 20-30 minutes. Gently wipe out ear with cotton swab to get all the ear wax out. Repeat if needed.

48) Apple Cider Vinegar for Ear Infection

Ingredients:
1 tsp apple cider vinegar (unfiltered)
2 Tbsp extra virgin olive oil
Clean towel, washcloth and eyedropper

Directions:
Mix both in saucepan until warm stirring well. Make sure it isn't too hot. Poor into eyedropper. Lay down with towel under your head with bad ear facing up. Fill ear with a few drops and leave in for 10 minutes. Place washcloth over ear and turn over so your head is on the towel and the ear drains onto the cloth. Repeat twice a day until infection subsides. If it doesn't go away within a few days, consult a doctor.

49) Turmeric for Toothache

Turmeric is used by many as a natural toothache treatment. It is an herb known for its pain-relieving abilities and possesses anti-bacterial and antiseptic properties. Just a teaspoon of turmeric powder in a small amount of purified water is enough to make a healing paste, which can be applied to the area or applied on a cotton ball, to be placed in your mouth. The turmeric can also be mixed with honey to sweeten.

50) Potato Compress for Eye Stye

Ingredients:

1 small potato, peeled and chopped

Sterile cloth

Directions:

Using a food processor or by hand, mash potato and make paste, spread it on a cloth and warm it in the microwave. Test that it is not too hot, apply it on inflamed eye to reduce swelling. Apply 3 times a day for 15 minutes.

51) Turmeric Compress for Eye Stye

Ingredients:

1 tsp ground turmeric

2 cup water

Finely woven straining cloth

Eyedropper

Directions:

Add turmeric to water and boil it until it reduces to half. Let cool and strain it several times until all granules are removed. Pour into eyedropper to use for eye drops 2-3 times a day until stye is gone.

52) Calendula Cure for Conjunctivitis (Pink Eye)

Ingredients:

1 tsp milk

1 tsp dried calendula flowers

1 cup water
Fine mesh strainer
Eyedropper
Sterile cloth

Directions:
Fill eyedropper with milk and place 5 drops into affected eye. Add calendula to cup of hot water and steep for 5 minutes. Strain into another cup and cool. Wash affected eye with clean cloth dipped into solution up to 4 times a day until it subsides.

53) Cucumber Relief for Dry Eyes

Ingredients:
1 small bowl warm water
4 drops lavender essential oil
2 cucumber slices (or raw potato slices)
Sterile cloth

Directions:
Add lavender oil to bowl of warm water, stir and dip cloth into water, squeeze excess water out and place over closed eyes for 5 minutes. Remove cloth and place cucumber slices on closed eyes for 5 minutes. Remove cucumbers and dip cloth into warm water with lavender oil again, drain excess water and wipe closed eyes. Repeat this every time your eyes feel dry.

54) Rose Petal Compress for Tired Eyes

Ingredients:
2-3 rose petals
1 cup water
Sterile cloth or cotton balls

Directions:
Bring water to boil, add rose pedals and steep for 10 minutes. Strain and cool. Soak cloth or cotton balls and place over closed eyelids to sooth tired or irritated eyes.

Home Remedies for Hair Problems

55) Hot Oil Treatment for Damaged or Dry Hair

Ingredients:

1/2 cup extra virgin olive oil

2-3 drops of your favorite essential oil (orange blossom, rose, or jasmine are good choices)

Directions:

Mix oils in a glass jar and store for 24 hours in a cool dark place. Warm it for just a few seconds by placing in a pan of warm water just before using. Make sure oil is lukewarm and apply to damp hair. Massage into scalp and work through the ends of hair. Wrap head with a plastic shower cap for at least 30 minutes. Rinse hair thoroughly and shampoo as usual. Use twice a month for best results. You can also use olive oil as a conditioner.

56) Olive Oil Leave-in Conditioner for Damaged Hair

Ingredients:

Extra virgin olive oil

Directions:

After shampooing hair, apply a few drops of olive oil to the palm of one hand, rub hands together to warm up oil, apply to damp hair and work into the ends. Do not rinse. If it feels to thick or your hair is very fine, add equal part of jojoba oil for a lighter treatment. This is a great way to repair damaged or frizzy hair and it even works to kill lice. So next time the kids bring home those nasty bugs from school, try applying a thick layer of olive oil to the whole head. It's a big money saver.

57) Lemon for Dandruff

Ingredients:

1 lemon

Directions:

Be a lemon head and cut a lemon in half. Rub the two halves into the scalp, leave for 10 minutes, then shampoo. Repeat a few times a week until dandruff disappears.

58) Apple Cider Vinegar for Dandruff

Ingredients:

1 cup apple cider vinegar

Directions:

Before shampooing, rinse hair with cider. Wrap head in a towel and leave for 30 minutes. Rinse completely and shampoo. Repeat 3 times a week until the dandruff is gone.

Remedies for Other Head-Related Issues

59) Basil for Vertigo/Dizziness

Ingredients:

1 tsp ground basil
1 tsp ground coriander seeds
1 cup hot water

Directions

Add ground basil and ground coriander seeds to a cup of hot water, let it steep for 5 minutes. Drink up to 4 times a day for relief.

60) Peppermint Tea for Dry Mouth

Ingredients:

1 Tbsp dried peppermint
1 Tbsp dried rosemary
1 cup hot water

Directions:

Add dried peppermint and rosemary to hot water, steep for 5 minutes. Using a mesh strainer, strain into another cup. Drink up to 4 times a day to treat dry mouth.

Chapter 5: Home Remedies for Skin Issues

The largest organ in the body is our skin and it is responsible for protecting all our internal organs. It acts as a barrier from foreign organisms of bacteria and viruses, so it is important to keep it healthy and the below remedies will help.

Home Remedies for Rashes, Itches, Burns & Bites

61) Coconut Oil Rub for Rashes/Thrush

Ingredients:

2 Tbsp coconut oil

1 tsp baking soda

Directions:

Mix to form a paste to apply on rash for 5 minutes, wash with warm water. Repeat daily until rash subsides. Coconut oil can also be used to treat thrush in babies when used by itself by putting some on your finger and applying to the tongue.

62) Licorice & Garlic for Shingles

Ingredients:

2 garlic cloves

1 tsp licorice powder

1 tsp or less of water

Directions:

Crush garlic with mortar and pestle. Add licorice powder and small amount of water to form paste. Apply to the area for 5 minutes and then wash with warm water. Use up to twice a day until shingles subside.

63) Peppermint Rub Remedy for Itching

Ingredients:

1 tsp dried peppermint

1 tsp dried basil

1 tsp or less of water

Directions:

Using a mortar, crush dried ingredients and mix with water to form a paste. Rub paste on the itchy area for 2 minutes and then wash with a gentle soap and warm water. Do this as soon as you get an itch instead of scratching it.

64) Oatmeal Soak for Psoriasis/Eczema

Ingredients:

1 cup apple cider vinegar (unfiltered)

1 cup colloidal oatmeal

Directions:

Grind the oatmeal in a coffee grinder, add to a hot bath with apple cider vinegar and soak in it for up to 30 minutes. Be careful getting out of the tub as it may be slippery. Pat yourself dry. Use up to 3 times per week until symptoms subside.

65) Milk Soak for Psoriasis

Ingredients:

1 milk

2 tsp extra virgin olive oil

Bag balm

Directions:

Mix and add to a warm bath and soak for 30 minutes. Use every day and then apply bag balm to area until psoriasis subsides. It will also help to avoid tomatoes, caffeine, and pork products.

66) Milk & Oil for Dry Skin

Ingredients:

1-2 tsp extra virgin olive oil

1/2 cup milk, warmed

Directions:

Apply extra virgin olive oil to the dry skin for 30 minutes. Soak a cloth in warm milk and apply the soaked cloth to the dry skin for 5 minutes. Wash clean with warm water. Do daily until it subsides.

67) Home Remedies for Eczema

Make a rice-flour hot compress to apply to the affected area and apply a mixture of 1 teaspoon camphor and 1 teaspoon sandalwood paste on the rashes.

Eating lots of asparagus will help promote the elimination of toxins and is considered a liver tonic because of its high amino acid content. Drink the water from the steamed asparagus. Also drinking the juice of cabbage that has anti-bacterial properties promotes healing. Watercress is said to keep eczema away with a daily drink made from spinach, celery, parsley and wheat grass.

68) Relief from Bed Bug Bites

Ingredients:
2-3 Tbsp white vinegar
5 drops of witch hazel oil

Directions:
Soak a cotton ball in white vinegar and add witch hazel oil to the cotton ball. Dab the bed bug bites with the soaked cotton ball. Use up to 2 times per day until the bed bug bites have healed.

69) Home Remedies for Burns

Ingredients:
Plain yogurt
Apple cider vinegar (unfiltered)
2 tsp lemon juice
1 tsp honey (optional)
1 cup water
1 tsp peppermint or lavender essential oil
1 tsp extra virgin olive oil

Directions:
Immediately after getting a small burn, apply yogurt to cool it. Wipe off after a few minutes and apply apple cider vinegar. Make lemon tea to help in calming and pain relief. After 20 minutes or so, mix oils and apply to area to ease the stinging sensation.

70) Soothing Remedy for Sunburn

Ingredients:

2 Tbsp apple cider vinegar (unfiltered)

2 Tbsp coconut oil

Directions:

Mix apple cider vinegar with coconut oil. Apply the mixture to the affected skin part. Continue using on the affected skin until it is back to its normal condition which may take a few days.

71) Heal Poison Ivy with Apple Cider Vinegar

To soothe itch and the burning caused by the poison ivy, dampen cotton balls or Q-tips by dipping them in apple cider vinegar and dabbing on the affected areas and then let dry. Dab again. Be sure to use small amounts on the affected areas as using too much can cause a more painful burn.

Home Remedy for Facial Skin Cleanser/Wrinkles

72) Honey & Baking Soda Facial Scrub

Ingredients:

1/2 Tbsp raw honey

1 Tbsp baking soda

1 drop frankincense (Boswellia) essential oil

1 drop lavender essential oil

1 drop geranium essential oil

Directions:

Mix honey and baking soda and add essential oils. Take a warm towel and place it on your face to open the pores before applying scrub.

73) Kiwi Facial Scrub

Ingredients:

1 Tbsp sweet almond oil

2 Tbsp cane sugar

1/2 kiwi, minced

Directions:

Mix together the oil and sugar, add kiwi. Mix well and apply with circular motion massaging the face and neck for at least 3 minutes. Rinse well with warm water and apply face moisturizer. To keep scrub stored, cover and keep in the fridge for up to two weeks.

74) Aloe Vera & Olive Oil for Wrinkles

Ingredients:

1 Tbsp aloe vera gel

1 Tbsp extra virgin olive oil

Directions:

Massage aloe vera gel into wrinkles. Leave on for 15 minutes. Then massage olive oil into wrinkles and leave for 15 minutes. Wash clean with warm water. Use 2 times a day for as long as wanted.

Home Remedies for Acne

75) Avocado and Tomatoes for Acne

Avocado contains plenty of vitamins A, C, E and B complex, which are all essential for good skin. It also has strong anti-bacterial and anti-fungal properties, so makes an excellent treatment for acne or any other irritating skin conditions. Make up a paste of avocado pulp and apply to skin once or twice a day for 30 minutes. Ripe tomatoes also are good for acne. Smash a ripe tomato and apply to skin for an hour. Rinse with warm water.

76) Cinnamon Honey for Acne

Ingredients:

2 Tbsp baking soda

1 tsp cinnamon

2 Tbsp lemon juice

5 Tbsp Manuka honey

Directions:

Mix all well in a bowl and apply to the acne for 5 minutes and then wash it clean with warm water. Use once a day until acne subsides. Baking soda exfoliates your skin, unblocking pores and removes dead skin. Cinnamon is an antioxidant that helps repair the damage caused by acne. Manuka honey helps by reducing the buildup of bacteria in your pores and preventing inflammation. Lemon juice helps by drying out and disinfecting the skin.

Other Skin Home Remedies

77) Black Tea & Garlic Paste for Cold Sores

Ingredients:

1 tsp dried black tea leaves

1 clove garlic

1 tsp or less water

Directions:

Crush tea leaves and garlic using mortar and pestle. Mix with a small amount of water to make a paste to apply to cold sore for 15 minutes. Wash clean with warm water. Use every 2-3 hours until sore is healed.

78) Green Tea Leaves for Blackheads

Ingredients:

1 tsp dry green tea leaves

5 drops of tea tree oil

Directions:

Crush green tea leaves using a mortar and pestle and mix with a small amount of water to form a paste. Add 5 drops of tea tree oil to the paste. Gently rub the paste into the blackheads and leave for 2 minutes. Wash clean with warm water. Repeat daily until skin is clear.

79) Apple Cider Vinegar for Wart Remover

File down the warts and clean the skin around it. Apply petroleum jelly to the skin around the warts to prevent the cider from burning the skin. Dampen a cotton ball with cider and place it on the wart covering it up and placing a band aid to hold it. Leave the cotton ball on overnight. Repeat the process for 5 days until wart is gone.

80) Apple Cider Vinegar to Heal Varicose Veins

Varicose veins are usually developed in the legs and is immediately caused by poor blood circulation. Because Apple cider vinegar improves circulation, it can help relieve the symptoms of varicose veins like pain, cramps, heaviness, tingling itching and swelling.

Ingredients:

1/2 cup apple cider vinegar (unfiltered)

1/2 raw carrot

3 Tbsp aloe vera gel

Directions:

Add all to blender to make a creamy paste. Massage the affected area vigorously. Also, you can use a sterile gauze moistened with apple cider vinegar and keep it in place on top of the varicose veins for a few minutes. Alternate these two for best results.

Chapter 6: Home Remedies for Hypertension

If you have hypertension, otherwise known as high blood pressure, your doctor may want you to take medication because high blood pressure is serious and can lead to heart disease. Before getting on medication, it can be beneficial to try some home remedies since medication can have harsh side effects. Tell your doctor what you plan on trying. Depending on how high your blood pressure is will determine if your doctor approves. He may ask you to take your blood pressure every day if he approves. I am giving you several home remedies to try since everyone is different and high blood pressure is nothing to ignore but if it gets dangerously high, you should contact your doctor. If one remedy doesn't lower it within a few weeks, try another.

The first one below was faithfully used by my grandmother to control her blood pressure. She didn't need medication and her doctor was amazed at how well it worked.

Remedies for Lowering Blood Pressure

81) Apple Cider Vinegar & Garlic to Lower Blood Pressure

Ingredients:
1/2 cup apple cider vinegar (unfiltered)
3 garlic cloves, minced

Directions:
Mix together in a mason jar and let sit for about 3 days before using. Add 2 tablespoons to water or make as a tea every day (these measurements can be adjusted according to the strength desired). Stored in refrigerator it will last approximately a week when taking it every day.

Consuming apple cider vinegar can help lower triglycerides, the main elements of natural fats and oil and will lower blood pressure considerably.

82)Lemons to Lower Blood Pressure

Ingredients:

1/2 fresh lemon, juiced

1 cup water

Directions:

Add lemon juice to warm water and drink every morning on an empty stomach. Do not add salt or sugar for best results.

83)Garlic & Milk to Lower Blood Pressure

Ingredients:

1-2 crushed garlic cloves

1 cup milk

Directions:

Crush fresh garlic cloves and add to milk to drink every day.

84)Onions to Lower Blood Pressure

Ingredients:

1 medium size raw onion

1 tsp honey

1 cup water

Directions:

Eat onion raw every day or crush to make 1/2 tsp of onion juice, add honey to warm water. Drink twice a day for 1-2 weeks for results. Onions have an antioxidant flavanol called quercetin that lowers blood pressure.

85)Lower Blood Pressure with Honey

Three more ways to use honey to reduce blood pressure are:

1) 2 tsp on empty stomach each morning.

2) Mix 1 tsp honey and 1 tsp ginger juice with 2 tsp cumin seed powder. Eat twice a day.

3) Mix 1 tsp each of basil juice and honey to take on empty stomach daily.

86) Fenugreek Seeds to Lower Blood Pressure

Ingredients:

1-2 tsp fenugreek seeds

1 cup water

Directions:

Add seeds to water and let sit for 2 minutes. Strain and put seeds in blender to make a paste. Eat once every morning on empty stomach and once in the evening for 2-3 months.

87) Blueberry & Honey to Lower Blood Pressure

Ingredients:

8 Tbsp dried blueberries

4 cups water

1 cup honey

Glass jar with airtight lid that will hold 2 cups

Directions:

Add the dried berries to water, simmer over low heat until reduced by half. Strain and press to extract juice. Pour the liquid back into the pot and stir in the honey blending together thoroughly. Once mixed, bottle and store in the refrigerator for up to 3-4 weeks. Use as a tea or simply take 1 tablespoon twice daily.

88) Watermelon Seeds to Lower Blood Pressure

Ingredients:

2 tsp crushed watermelon seeds

1 cup water

Directions:

Add crushed seeds to boiled water and steep for 1 hour. Strain and drink 4 tablespoons at a time throughout the day.

89) Cat's Claw Lowers Blood Pressure

Ingredients:

2 Tbsp dried cats claw

2 cups water

1-2 tsp honey or lemon

Directions:

Bring the cat's claw and water to a slow simmer covered over low heat for 40-45 minutes. Add more water if too concentrated. Strain and add honey and/or lemon. Drink once a day.

90) Other Foods that Lower Blood Pressure

There are several foods that help in lowering blood pressure. You can use your imagination and make up teas, snacks, salads, and whole meals with a combination of the foods listed below:

- Bananas – eat 1-2 a day
- Berries such as blueberries, strawberries, raspberries
- Carrots – eat 2 or 3 raw carrots a day
- Cayenne pepper – add to salads, soups or entrees
- Celery – eat a stalk with a glass of water every day
- Coconut – drink a glass of coconut water every day, cook with coconut oil
- Dark chocolate – eat 100 grams a day
- Dried apricots – eat a few every day
- Fatty fish such as salmon and mackerel – 2-3 times a week
- Herbal teas that contain hibiscus
- Orange juice – drink a glass every morning
- Red beets – make juice from them or cook
- Spinach and other leafy greens – use fresh in salads
- Sweet potatoes – bake 1 with skin on to eat every day
- Zucchini – add to salads and dishes

Chapter 7: Alleviating Allergies/Asthma

If you are under the care of a doctor for allergies, asthma or hay fever and taking medication, be sure to discuss taking these remedies prior to trying them as you shouldn't take both.

Combat Seasonal Allergies with Home Remedies

91) Apple Cider Vinegar for Allergies

Ingredients:

2 tsp apple cider vinegar (unfiltered)

1 tsp honey

1 cup water

Directions:

Bring water to boiling, add apple cider vinegar and honey. Stir and drink once in the morning and once at night every day that allergies are bothering you. Apple cider vinegar mainly acts to balance the pH level of the body which helps issues like allergies. It also helps boost the immune system.

92) Tomato Juice Tea for Allergy Relief

Ingredients:

1 cup of tomato juice

1/2 tsp of hot sauce (optional)

1 tsp of freshly chopped garlic.

1 tsp of lemon juice

Small pinch of celery salt

Directions:

Mix all and heat well. Drink twice daily for allergies. This recipe can help open clogged nasal passages to make breathing a little easier. The tomato juice and lemon are high in nutrients that help to support your immune system.

93) Nettle Leaf & Peppermint Allergy Remedy

Ingredients:

1 Tbsp dried nettle leaf

1 Tbsp dried peppermint

1 cup water

Directions:

Bring water to boil, add dried nettle leaf and peppermint to hot water and let it steep for 5 minutes. Strain the water into another cup using a fine mesh strainer. Drink up to 4 times per day until the allergy symptoms subside. Nettle leaf acts as a antihistamine and peppermint is an effective decongestant that can unplug your nose and also relieve any inflammation you may have.

94) Lavender & Eucalyptus Oil for Asthma

Ingredients:

10 drops lavender oil

10 drops eucalyptus oil

Directions:

Put 5 drops of each oil on a paper towel and place it on your pillow before going to sleep and sleep with it all night. Upon waking, throw it away. Add 5 drops of each oil to a bowl of boiling water and breathe in the steam with deep breaths for 5 minutes. Repeat each day until symptoms subside.

95) Fig Tea for Asthma

Ingredients:

3-4 dried figs

1/4 lemon

1 cup water

Directions:

Slice a lemon into quarters, add one quarter of a lemon and figs to the water and soak overnight. Eat the figs the next morning on an empty stomach. You can also make tea out of liquid.

There are ingredients in figs that help promote respiratory health and help asthma symptoms to dissipate. It has been shown that those suffering from asthma do not get enough vitamin C so taking lemon may help as they are rich in vitamin C, which may help reduce asthma symptoms. Lemon contains some antioxidants that help calm down the inflammation of the internal lining of the respiratory tract, relieving the symptoms associated with asthma. If you have asthma, try using lemon in as much as possible.

96) Garlic Remedy for Sinusitis

Ingredients:
10 drops oregano oil
3 cloves of garlic
Bowl of hot water

Directions:
Put 5 drops of oregano oil on a paper towel and place it on your pillow and sleep with it all night. Upon waking, throw it away. Add 3 cloves of garlic and 5 drops oregano oil to a bowl of boiling water and breathe in the steam with deep breaths for 5 minutes. Repeat each day until symptoms subside.

Home Remedies for Hay Fever

Hay fever is otherwise known as allergic rhinitis. It is an allergy to the pollen that is released by grasses, flowers, and trees. Allergy season is usually in the spring and fall. Histamines are released when these pollens are inhaled or just smelled. House dust mites, pet dander or bird feathers can also cause the watery eyes, running or stuffy tickling nose, sneezing, itchy throat and sometimes hives. Many home remedies above that help allergies or asthma can help with hay fever, plus here are some other remedies. If you are under the care of a doctor for allergies or hay fever and taking medication, be sure to discuss taking these remedies prior to trying them.

Ingredients:

1 Tbsp elderflower heads

1-1/2 cups brown sugar

3 lemons, sliced

2 oranges, sliced

3 pints hot water

3-1/2 Tbsp tartaric acid (or 6 Tbsp cream of tartar)

Directions:

Bring water to boil, mix all together into hot water, steep in covered bowl for 24 hours. Strain into a pan and bring to boil until sugar is dissolved. Cool and store in covered bottle in refrigerator or freezer. Heat and drink a cup whenever hay fever hits. If you don't have access to elderflowers, you can substitute with elderberry syrup.

98) Other Remedies for Hay Fever

- Add a teaspoon of local honey and 6-8 drops of apple cider vinegar to a cup of hot water and drink in the morning. Start before the season starts and then increase the amount of honey as it progresses.
- Stay inside on hot and windy days so it is best to stay inside during this time. Pollen settles after dark throughout the night into early morning and you should also stay inside then
- Apply Vaseline to inside of nose to reduce irritation.
- Before bed take a shower and wash hair to remove any pollen that may irritate you during the night.
- Stay away from a lot of sugar, flour, dairy products and salt during the season but eat lots of fish, hot soups, fruits and vegetables except for acidy ones like tomatoes or citrus.
- Using a vaporizer with your favorite aromatherapy oil helps clear nasal passages.
- A popular remedy for hay fever is green tea as it contains oxidants and helps treat allergies and prevent infections.

Chapter 8: Remedies for Other Common Ailments

There are so many illnesses and health problems but there is a home remedies for just about anything you have. Below are some I have used as well as others collected from difference resources for common complaints such as cramps, urinary tract infections (UTIs), constipation, heartburn, and other gastrointestinal problems as well as sleeping problems.

Home Remedies for Women's Complaints

99) Relief for Monthly Menstrual Cramps

Ingredients:

30 ml gin

1 Tbsp honey

Directions:

Mix well and drink when needed for menstrual cramps.

100)   Raspberries for Women's Health

Ingredients:

2-3 tsp dried red raspberry leaf (or 2-3 Tbsp fresh raspberries)

1 cup water

1 tsp honey or lemon

Directions:

Bring water to a boil, add raspberry leaves, let steep for 6-8 minutes. Strain well, add honey and lemon to taste. Not only will this help cramps but will be a good tea to have every day for great muscle health including your heart and other organs.

101)   Baking Soda for UTIs

Ingredients:

1 tsp baking soda

1 cup water

Directions:

Dissolve baking soda in water and drink the whole thing first thing in the morning. If you are trying to avoid salt, don't use for more than a few days. Drink extra water during the day and plenty of 100% cranberry or blueberry juice without added sugar.

102)   Parsley Leaves for UTIs

Ingredients:

1 cup fresh parsley leaves or 2 Tbsp dried

1-2 cups water

Directions:

Using fresh parsley is best. Add it to water, boil and then simmer for 10 minutes. Strain leaves and drink as a hot tea or cool and have iced tea. If using dried leaves, place in hot water, cover and steep for 8 minutes, strain and drink twice a day until symptoms subside. If you get UTIs often, avoid citrus, chocolate, carbonated drinks and caffeine. If this doesn't do the trick, see your doctor.

103)   Lemon and Cream of Tartar for UTIs

Ingredients:

1-1/2 cream of tartar cup

1/2 cup warm water

1 tsp lemon or lime juice to taste

Directions:

Stir cream of tartar into warm water, add juice to flavor and drink 1-2 times a day. Drink it on a regular basis to keep UTIs away.

Home Remedies for Gastrointestinal Issues

104)   Ginger for Bloating and Flatulence

Ingredients:

1 tsp freshly grated ginger or 2 tsp ginger juice

1 tsp honey

1-1/2 cups water

Directions:

Bring water to boil, add ginger and simmer for 10 minutes. Strain, add honey and cool to drink twice a day.

105)   *Peppermint for Lactose Intolerance*

Ingredients:

1 tsp dried peppermint leaves

1 cup water

Directions:

Bring water to boil, add peppermint leaves, cover and simmer for 10 minutes. Strain and drink twice a day to relieve symptoms. You can also add peppermint leaves to salads or other dishes. Also helps other intestinal issues.

106)   *Apple Cider Vinegar for Indigestion, Gas, Stomachache*

Ingredients:

1 Tbsp apple cider vinegar (unfiltered)

1 tsp raw honey

1 cup water

Directions:

Bring water to boil, add apple cider vinegar and honey and drink 2-3 times a day to reduce symptoms and maintain a healthy digestive system.

107)   *Aloe Vera for Acid Reflux or Heartburn*

Ingredients:

1 ounce Aloe Vera syrup

Directions:

Drink by itself or poured into a juice that doesn't normally upset your stomach before each meal and at any time you feel indigestion, heartburn or acid reflux. Within a few weeks, you may not need it. However, if severe symptoms persist see your doctor.

Other remedies for heartburn are pickle juice (and a pickle), 2 tsp apple cider vinegar in a glass of water or swallowing a teaspoon of mustard seeds without chewing them with a glass of water.

108)   Honey and Apples to Stop Diarrhea

Ingredients:

4 Tbsp honey

1 Tbsp apple cider vinegar (unfiltered)

1 cup water

1/2 cup unsweetened applesauce

2 slices of wheat toast

Directions:

Bring water to boil, add honey and apple cider, stir and let cool. Drink 2-3 times a day until symptoms subside. Spread applesauce on toast or eat separately and have with your tea once a day. Apples have pectin which is known to firm up stool and ease diarrhea.

109)   Flaxseed as a Laxative

Ingredients:

1 8 oz. glass of orange juice with pulp

1 Tbsp flaxseed oil

Directions:

Mix together and drink for results within about 5 hours.

110)   Dandelions are Dandy for Constipation

Ingredients:

1-2 dried dandelion leaves

1 cup water heated

Directions:

Place leaves in a cup and pour hot water over them and steep for 8-10 minutes. Drink up to 3 times a day until you get relief. This is a gentle laxative good for inactive persons.

111) Oil to Get You Going Potty

Ingredients:

1 tsp lemon juice

1 Tbsp extra virgin olive oil

Directions:

This works best on an empty stomach, so have a tablespoon of olive oil with lemon juice added before you eat anything else in the morning. If you forget, wait until you haven't eaten for a while. Lemon juice also acts as a natural aid for constipation. Children can take this remedy if you can get them to swallow it. It's better than castor oil that us old folks had to take. Add a little honey to help.

112) Get Relief with Blackstrap Molasses

Ingredients:

1 tsp blackstrap molasses

1 cup water or tea

Directions:

Add molasses to warm water and drink in the morning before eating. You can use any flavor of tea if molasses flavor is too much for you. Increase the amount of molasses up to 2 tablespoons if a teaspoon doesn't do the job but increase the amount slowly so you don't have an accident.

Home Remedies for Stones

113) Celery to Ease Kidney Stones

Ingredients:

1 glass of celery juice or 1-2 tsp celery seeds

Directions:

Drink celery juice as much as possible along with lots of water to ease the pain of stones and as a diuretic to flush them out. Make tea from celery seeds to help pass kidney stones and help with high blood pressure or gout.

114)   *Apple Cider Vinegar for Kidney Stones*

Ingredients:

2 tsp apple cider vinegar (unfiltered)

1 tsp honey

1 cup water

Directions:

Bring water to boiling, add apple cider vinegar and honey. Stir and drink 3-4 times a day if you have stones. Drink once a day as a preventative measure to keep them from forming.

115)   *Kidney Beans for the Kidneys*

Ingredients:

1 cup of dried kidney beans

Sprinkle of salt for taste

Directions:

Clean beans of any debris, wash beans and place in pot to bring to a boil, then turn down heat and simmer for two hours or until soft and tender. Strain liquid and cool and then strain again. Drink all the broth within a day. Storing it over 24 hours will make it lose its therapeutic properties. You can use the beans in a stew or salad.

116)   *Wheatgrass for Kidney Stones and Detoxing*

Ingredients:

1 tsp lemon juice

1 tsp basil juice

1 8 oz glass wheatgrass juice

Directions:

Mix all well and drink 2-3 times a day to treat stones. Wheatgrass stimulates urine flow to help pass stones and has nutrients to help detox and cleanse kidneys.

117)   Juice Cocktail for Gallstones

Ingredients:

2 raw carrots, peeled

1 raw beet, peeled

1 raw cucumber, peeled

1 pear, peeled

1 celery stalk (or ½ cup of celery juice)

1 cup St. John's Wart tea from 4-5 leaves

1/2 cup lemon juice

1 tsp turmeric

1 tsp honey (optional)

Directions:

Make St. John's Wart tea by boiling a cup of water with leaves and strain. Put all in blender and blend until you have juice. Drink 2 times a day for two weeks or until symptoms of gallstones subside.

Home Remedies for Sleeping Problems

118)   Cherries and Vanilla to Help You Sleep

Ingredients:

6-8 ounces tart cherry juice (it must be tart)

1-2 drops vanilla extract

Directions:

Drink just the tart cherry juice first thing in the morning. At night about an hour before bed, add vanilla to the same amount help relax you. Tart cherry juice has melatonin to regulate sleep.

119)   Chamomile Lavender Tea for Insomnia

Ingredients:

1 tsp lavender buds

1 tsp chamomile buds

1 cup water

Honey or milk to taste

Directions:

Bring water to boil, add lavender and chamomile buds, steep for 10 to 15 minutes. Strain and add a little honey and/or milk

120) Let Sweet Milk Put You to Sleep

Ingredients:

1 glass milk

2-4 tsp honey

1/4 tsp nutmeg

Directions:

Warm up milk to almost boiling, add honey and nutmeg and let cool to drinking temperature. Drink 30 minutes before bedtime.

Chapter 9: Home Remedy Glossary

Many common spices, herbs, fruits, vegetables, and juices found in your kitchen are used in this book for home remedies of all kinds. As a cross reference, most items included in recipes that may not be familiar or that may be familiar but have powerful uses that you may not have known before are listed below alphabetically.

Also included for many of these is what they are best known to be remedies for so that if you need to know what a certain substance is good for, you can easily look it up here. You can even get creative and come up with some recipes of your own by putting items from the glossary together. Also, Chapter 10 is an index of ingredients showing what pages they appear on, so you can find them easily.

May you find items that are beneficial to you and your family. Wishing you the best health on your home remedy journey.

Alfalfa/Alfalfa Leaves: Alfalfa can be used for bladder and prostate conditions, kidney conditions, and helps increase urine flow. It can also be used for high cholesterol, osteoarthritis, rheumatoid arthritis, diabetes, upset stomach, and asthma.

Almonds/Almond Oil: Almonds have important micronutrients and are effective in dealing with bronchitis and other respiratory tract problems. They are a source of potassium and magnesium to boost the immune system and prevent respiratory infections. Almond oil is good for treating inflammation, skin issues such as eczema, psoriasis, and dermatitis or dry skin.

Aloe Vera: Aloe Vera is among the best herbal remedies for skin problems due to its cooling and soothing properties. The pulp of this plant helps prevent redness and inflammation of the skin. Aloe extracts act as a skin cleanser removing impurities, including bacteria. Directly apply the pulp of the aloe leaf to the skin, let it stay for a few minutes, and then rinse off.

any other home health remedy. It is made from apple cider that has been fermented like any other vinegar. When using for home remedies, you should use the diluted raw and unfiltered apple cider vinegar. It contains acetic acids, which have an alkaline effect on the body and balances the pH levels that can reduce the risk of chronic illnesses by mixing 1 to 2 teaspoons to 8 ounces of water, drinking before meals and rinsing mouth after drinking to protect tooth enamel from the acetic acid.

One 2007 study found that two tablespoons of apple cider vinegar can lower blood sugar levels in those with type 2 diabetes. Studies also show that apple cider vinegar can lower cholesterol and triglyceride levels, and other heart disease risk factors. It can also boost gut health, fight fungal infections, treat seasonal allergies, benefit weight loss, enhance circulation, and reduce heartburn and acid reflux. Apple cider vinegar is filled with enzymes, vitamins and minerals when you drink it raw. Detoxifying with it has great benefits to the aging process and removes all the toxins collected in the body that the body's natural detoxifying process is not able to flush out. It is believed to help detoxify and cleanse the liver. It can be helpful to protect your liver while on medications or when withdrawing from prescription drugs.

Apple Cider Vinegar contains a type of acid that promotes the growth of probiotics that help eliminate yeasts from the system. Consume 1 tablespoon of vinegar three times daily and remove sugar from your diet. Apple Cider Vinegar may be good for the stomach because it introduces more acids to the digestive tract. The acid also fights several types of bacteria as an anti-microbial agent.

Apple Cider Vinegar lowers glucose and insulin levels and helps in weight loss. It also increases satiety and lowers the appetite urging the body to burn stored calories. Apple Cider Vinegar also has acids and enzymes that raise body metabolism and burn body fat. It also reduces water retention working well for edema.

If it irritates your throat, make salad dressing with olive oil and have in everyday on a salad. Dressing can be made using three parts olive oil to one part or more of apple cider vinegar depending on your taste with seasonings or lemon for added flavor.

Besides using it for home health remedies, apple cider vinegar can be used as an antibacterial cleaner by diluting a half a cup of apple cider vinegar with 1 cup of water and putting in a spray bottle to use to clean bathroom or kitchen surfaces, windows or mirrors and then wiping with a cloth for a shiny finish.

Avocado: Avocados are a fruit native to Mexico and the Aztecs thought of the avocado as the fruit of fertility and believed it had aphrodisiac properties. It has a good amount of Vitamin E that can be good for lowering cholesterol. Because of its Vitamin A, B6, and folic acid it is considered good for controlling diabetes and helps rheumatoid arthritis. It helps improve intestinal problems, improves vision and has beauty applications since it slows aging of the skin and keeps hair silky and shiny.

Bag Balm: Bag Balm is a salve developed in 1899 to soothe cow udders after milking. It can be is used to treat chapped and irritated skin. It is made up of Petrolatum, Lanolin, Paraffin wax, and 8-Hydroxyquinoline Sulfate. After having it for some time, it may turn a darker color but will still have its properties and be effective. Most drug stores sell it.

Basil: Basil helps you feel more coordinated and alleviates many of the symptoms of vertigo. Basil is a powerful herb for the treatment of the worst forms of acne. Boiling the leaves of this herb in water and using the water as a face wash daily can help prevent formation of acne.

Bay Leaf: The ancient Greeks and Romans loved bay leaves. They used it to achieve clairvoyance, inspiration and happiness. Bay leaf may also act as an expectorant and soften the mucus that may have built up in the respiratory tract, thereby reducing the severity of symptoms associated with bronchitis.

Beets: Beets are a major source of phytochemicals and betalain pigments, a group of reddish pigments found in some fruits. One of Betalian pigments, betaine, is an active antioxidant, and anti-inflammatory. Consuming beets that are rich in betaine can help in increasing metabolism, improving the mechanism for insulin resistance, moods and discourage the activity of genes that hold fat. To consume beets as a juice, combine beets, a whole lemon, several apples, gingerroot and celery in a blender.

Bell Peppers: Bell peppers of all colors are a good remedy for pain. They contain an active enzyme known as capsaicin, which is thought to stimulate the release of endorphins (feel good hormones) of the body, which provides a natural analgesic action. Bell peppers are extremely versatile and can be added to almost any food that you like.

Black Beans: Black beans are rich in resistant-starches. Just like in raw oats, black beans contain a high level of resistant starches that serve as food for healthy digestive bacteria and ferment into butyrate, an inflammation-lessening fatty acid. Black beans can lower glucose and insulin levels after meals and effectively decrease inflammation.

Boswellia (Frankincense): Boswellia can be used to alleviate asthma and may have protective effects against diseases like leukemia and breast cancer. Boswellia has been used for well-being, skin disorders, infections, wound healing, joint problems, menstrual disorders, and bruises. Boswellia has been used to tone the skin and smooth wrinkles. Research has focused on its possible benefit for conditions such as arthritis, inflammatory bowel diseases, and asthma. Boswellia may also have anti-cancer effects. There is strong evidence to support the use of boswellia for osteoarthritis. There is good evidence to support its use for asthma and swelling in people who have brain tumors. Side effects may be upset of the stomach.

Broccoli: Broccoli is a heart-healthy food as it is rich in calcium, which is required for the optimum functioning of the heart. Eating broccoli everyday can cut down the risk of congestive heart failure and other heart conditions. Broccoli contains glucosinolate, a natural anti-inflammatory in pungent plants such as mustard, cabbage and horseradish. It was found to decrease the production mediators in the genetic level that promote inflammation. Broccoli is rich in Vitamin K, which helps regulate inflammatory responses in the body.

Bromelain: Bromelain is basically an enzyme that comes from pineapple. Bromelain is thought to be an excellent natural remedy for almost all types of pain and is thought to work by reducing the levels of prostaglandins in the body (the hormones that cause inflammation of tissues and induce pain). Bromelain is believed to be the best remedy when it comes to dealing with pain of the musculoskeletal system such as arthritis and general muscle pain as well as reducing inflammation in the whole body. It is also beneficial for asthma, autoimmune diseases, and digestive disorders. It can help to soothe the gut and reduce many of the worst symptoms of inflammatory bowel disease, such as diarrhea, stomach upset, bloating, and cramping. Bromelain is found in the core and stem of the pineapple and you can eat or press this for the juice to get the enzymatic mixture. If you blend pineapples and then strain out the concentrated juice, you can also get a healthy dose of these enzymes.

Cabbage: Cabbage can draw out toxins. You can also drink the juice of the cabbage sweetened with a teaspoon of honey along with a warm broth made from boiling onions with a touch of cinnamon or cloves to help open airway and reduce congestion. Cabbage can treat gout by cutting the center hard core out of cabbage leaves then use a meat hammer to beat cabbage leaves so juice starts to come out, place them on the effected joint and wrap an ace bandage around the joint.

Calendula: Calendula (calendula officinalis) flowers are best known as a skin remedy. The plants natural astringent and antibiotic properties make it great as a paste for healing minor wounds, skin ulcers, burns, sunburn, bruises, insect bites and stings. It can treat eczema or psoriasis, and diaper rash. As a tea it is good for detoxing, fever, cramps, stomachache, flu and colds.

Cat's Claw: Cat's Claw is a woody climbing vine found in South and Central America, with its most notable use being in the Amazon rainforest. It is named after the thorns on the plant which are hooked, much like cat's claws. It has been used as a traditional remedy in its native habitat for a long time, but test tube studies finally revealed evidence for promising benefits, one amongst them being lowering blood pressure. It does so by dilating the blood vessels (known as vasodilation) and therefore lowering the pressure by allowing blood to flow through more readily. It can also act as a mild diuretic, getting rid of unneeded salt and water in the body, which can again reduce hypertension. The tannins and flavonoid are most likely the main constituents that account for the herbs healing actions.

Catnip: Catnip may remind you of the effect it has on cats, but it has many medicinal uses for humans too. Catnip has the opposite effect on people that it does for cats. It has been used for thousands of years as a mild sedative, muscle relaxer, a digestive aid and can stimulate menstrual flow. Catnip (also known as Catmint or Field Balm) is a member of the mint family and is a perennial herb that is said to grow up to 3-4 feet.

Cayenne Pepper: Cayenne peppers contains high levels of capsaicin, which is a common ingredient in many topical pain relief creams. It is one of the most effective treatments for fighting back pain. Some other benefits of cayenne pepper include weight loss, good blood circulation, good digestion, lowers cholesterol and boosts immunity. It can function as a treatment for heart diseases, dyspepsia, inflammation, headaches, and throat congestion. They contain vitamin E, vitamin C, vitamin K, carotenoids and the complete B complex. It is also a source of calcium, potassium, manganese, and dietary fiber.

Cayenne Pepper Warning: Be careful when using cayenne pepper because excess consumption may cause burning sensations in the throat, stomach, or rectum. Like with any hot pepper, you should wear gloves when handling it as it is hard to wash off hands and if you happen to rub your eye after handling, you will have a burning eye for a while. If that happens, wash the hands with milk and then soak a paper towel in milk to pat on the eye and let it sit and soak into the eye. Milk works best because it breaks down the oil in the pepper. You can also wash eye out with saline solution but don't use water as it will just spread the hot oil.

Chamomile: Chamomile oils are commonly used for aromatherapy and it is believed that they possess remarkable relaxing and calming properties. It may reduce symptoms associated with fibromyalgia or anxiety, tension and insomnia.

Cherries: Cherries are natural anti-inflammatories, which are effective in lowering uric acid levels. High amounts of

antioxidants called anthocyanins are the key to the pain-fighting power of cherries and help ease arthritis and joint pain and inflammation. Pain-calming anthocyanins are also found in blackberries, raspberries, and strawberries.
Tart Cherries are incredibly rich in melatonin, the hormone responsible for regulating our sleep-wake cycles, so indulging in a glass of the tart but sweet ruby red liquid every morning and night will help you keep your sleep schedule on track.

Chia Seeds: One study found that increasing the doses of chia seeds can decrease the spikes in blood sugar level. The spikes in blood sugar levels after eating have been a suspected cause of inflammation due to the overproduction of free radicals called reactive oxygen species. Chia seeds can also enhance weight loss, reduce appetite and can help keep the body hydrated for a day. Chia seeds can be consumed as supplements or sprinkled on top of a dish or added to bread before baking.

Chili Pepper: There are many helpful medicinal uses of chili peppers. These peppers are rich in a compound known as capsaicin, which is thought to be a pain reliever. When applied topically, it is thought to reduce the secretion of neurochemicals that send pain signals to the brain, thereby reducing the pain and tenderness of the joints and other parts of the body.

Chlorella: Chlorella is thought to be effective in dealing with pain associated with fibromyalgia. Taking chlorella supplements can curb muscle pain and weakness, and boost energy levels. Chlorella is commercially available in most health food stores.

Chocolate Mint Leaves: Fresh mint herbs can relax your muscles, relieve sinus pressure, sooth a migraine, reduce flatulence, calm heartburn, relieve stomach of nausea or upset. This one is especially good because it has a chocolate flavor. Because mint has the chemical of menthol, it can be used to sooth chest and respiratory system problems.

Cinnamon: Cinnamon is one of the oldest spices from the bark of the cinnamon tree. It is rolled into sticks that are used for flavor and aroma in many dishes and drinks. It has been shown to lower blood sugar by increasing glucose metabolism and to improve capillary function and works to reduce the risk of diabetes or heart disease. This spice also has antimicrobial and anti-inflammatory effects to help fight colds and bacteria in your mouth, lower cholesterol, fight cancer, relieve stomachache, plus relieve joint and arthritis pain. It can be used for skin issues along with honey.

Coconut Water/Coconut Oil: Potassium helps keep fluid and electrolyte balance in the body, especially during exercise. Because there is more potassium than sodium in coconut water, the potassium may help balance out sodium's effect on blood pressure and possibly even help lower it. It also acts as a natural laxative and diuretic as it helps dilute urine as well as increase urine flow. Coconut water is also known as a healthy and digestive tonic.

Coriander Seeds: Coriander seeds are one of the most popular natural ingredients for fighting vertigo. Gargling with boiled coriander water can reduce and cure mouth ulcers. It can also be used as a cure for itchy skin and rashes by making a paste of coriander seeds with a little water and a teaspoon of honey. Apply paste on itchy skin for instant relief.

Cucumber: Cucumber is known to promote skin health and may also help deal with acne. Cucumis sativus, what we know as cucumber today, possesses many cooling and soothing properties, and is believed to purify the blood and the lymphatic system too. Drinking the juice of cucumber could therefore, help purify the blood and prevent acne caused due to blood disorders, and when applied topically, it can soothe damaged skin and reduce redness and inflammation.

Dandelion Leaves: Incredibly high in vitamins A and C, dandelion leaves can help repair damaged tissue and help clear the liver clear toxins out of the blood. Studies have shown anti-inflammatory properties due to the linoleic and linoleic acid. Linoleic is an essential fatty acid required by the body to produce prostaglandin-which basically regulates immune responses and suppresses inflammation. Because of its involvement with immune responses, dandelion shows great potential when it comes to treating rheumatoid arthritis. You can enjoy dandelion leaves in nice salad or brew tea with them.

Dark Chocolate: Cocoa is a chocolate powder made from roasted and ground cacao seeds. Cocoa powder contains polyphenols. Polyphenols are compounds found abundantly in plants. Several studies found that microbes in the stomach ferment chocolate anti-inflammatory compounds that stop the actions of genes connected to insulin resistance and inflammation. Eating dark chocolate is also healthy for the heart and can reduce blood sugar levels.

Elderflower/elderberries: Elderflowers are sweetly scented, creamy, white flowers from the elder tree that grow in clusters and appear in abundance in hedgerows and woodlands at the beginning of summer and make an aromatic cordial. Elder tree has berries that are high in immune-boosting compounds that help beat the cold and flu quickly. The elderberries contain Vitamins A, B, and C and stimulate the immune system. There are different varieties of elderberries: 1) Blue ones grow on west coast, 2) black ones mainly grow in the east, 3) red ones should be avoided as they can be toxic. You can find recipes for making syrup from the berries or flowers on the internet.

Eggs: Eggs are high in Vitamin D. Some studies have found that there is a relationship between Vitamin D deficiency and increase of inflammation. Though direct exposure to sunlight promotes the production of Vitamin D by the body, people nowadays are staying indoors more. To increase Vitamin D levels in the body, eating food rich in Vitamin D can help. Eggs help in keeping bones strong, fighting against depression and colds while reducing risks to certain cancers.

Eucalyptus Oil: Individuals suffering from bronchitis are often advised to try steam therapy to loosen the phlegm and make breathing easier. Adding a few drops of eucalyptus oil to your steam water could clear the obstructed airways of the lungs and reduce bacterial activity due to its antibacterial action and speeds up the healing process. Eucalyptus oil is a natural decongestant and helps to clear your airways, make breathing easier and prevent the buildup of mucus. Pure eucalyptus oil is believed to be a great help with asthma as it possesses valuable decongestant properties that make breathing easier. It also contains a chemical known as eucalyptol that makes breathing easier. Rubbing just a few drops of this oil on your sheets and bed covers can help you breathe in the aroma and get a good night's sleep.

Fenugreek seeds: Fenugreek seeds contain protein, vitamin C, niacin, potassium, and diosgenin (which is a compound that has properties similar to estrogen). Other active constituents in fenugreek are alkaloids, lysine and L-tryptophan, as well as steroidal saponins. They can help increase libido and lessen the effect of hot flashes and mood fluctuations that are common symptoms of menopause and PMS. They also have been used to treat arthritis, improve digestion, asthma, bronchitis, maintain a healthy metabolism, cure skin problems (wounds, rashes and boils), treat sore throat, and cure acid reflux. People who took 2 ounces (56g) of fenugreek seed each day lowered cholesterol by around 14 percent after 24 weeks and had lowered their risk of heart attack by more than 25 percent. The seeds can be sprinkled onto prepared food, or they can be consumed with water when in capsule form.

Flaxseed: Flaxseed or oil should be consumed by those with a plant-based diet and in need of an increased Omega-3 intake. It is more effective among females and particularly those who are currently experiencing menopause or are post-menopausal. Flax seeds should be consumed in relatively small portions throughout the day and they should be carefully considered by those with hypotension or thin blood, pregnant women and those on a plant-based diet who are deficient in iron. Ask your doctor if in doubt.

Garlic: Garlic contains allicin, a compound known to block enzymes that assist in bacterial and viral infections. Aged garlic extracts stimulate proteins that prevent inflammation while suppressing the signs of inflammation. Garlic can also help in fighting against colds and known for its efficiency in dealing with various heart-related conditions since centuries, and the ancient Egyptians have discovered more than 195 different uses of garlic! Several studies have found that taking raw garlic could help lower down elevated blood pressure levels and strengthening the heart tissue and preventing the worsening of symptoms. Like onions and leeks, it contains diallyl disulfide, an anti-inflammatory compound that limits the effects of pro-inflammatory cytokines. It can help fight the pain, inflammation and cartilage damage of arthritis. Garlic possesses wonderful anti-microbial and anti-bacterial properties that make it one of the best natural remedies for bronchitis. Consumption of garlic can prevent the growth of bacteria and viruses that cause the infection and may also help treat acute bronchitis. Chop a few cloves of garlic, boil them in some milk, and drink it before retiring to bed at night for relief.

Ginger: Ginger is often used as a natural remedy for common cold, and it turns out, it may also be effective against bronchitis. Ginger contains impressive immune-boosting properties and has excellent anti-inflammatory action that reduces swelling and congestion in the lungs and makes breathing easier for asthma. Ginger reduces inflammation in the digestive tract and can prevent and treat indigestion, helps prevent nausea and vomiting, reduce abdominal pain, stomach cramping, and other symptoms of gastric distress, reducing the risk of blood clots. It can prevent irregular heartbeat and has an anti-inflammatory effect on the cardiovascular system. It reduces memory impairment such as in Alzheimer's disease and reduces high blood pressure. Ginger has also been shown to improve circulation and has been used in Asian cultures for hundreds of years to treat cold hands and feet or Raynaud's disease. Gingerols are compounds that are anti-oxidants, anti-bacterial and anti-inflammatory.

Gingko Biloba: Ginkgo biloba is a tree that is known as a "living fossil" having remained unchanged for millions of years. It is so tough that it was the first tree to grow after the atomic bomb hit Hiroshima, where almost all other vegetation was destroyed. Gingko Biloba is a popular herb that is used to deal with a wide range of health conditions and disorders. It is believed that gingko can improve circulation and boost the function of the immune system, the brain, the libido and improves concentration for people with ADHD symptoms. It reduces fatigue and weakness associated with fibromyalgia and fights PMS. Benefits include improved cognitive function, positive mood, increased energy, and improved memory. It can help improve the flow of blood thus helping repair any damaged nerves or cells as in diabetes or other conditions with nerve damage.

Green tea: Green tea contains high concentrations of catechins, which are a type of flavonoid that has anti-oxidant and anti-inflammatory properties to protect the body from free radicals that start many diseases in the body. The most potent catechin called epigallocatechin gallate (EGCG) is found only in Green tea. It is also good in preventing the development and growth of skin tumors.

Honey: Honey is one of the oldest remedies known to man - the ancient Egyptians it was used for high blood pressure. Honey has been in use as a natural treatment for asthma and its symptoms. It was found that patients experiencing asthma symptoms could get relief after just inhaling the smell of honey! Honey is best taken before bed. Take one teaspoon with some cinnamon powder which helps remove phlegm to let you to sleep better.

Kiwi: Kiwi is a fruit that contains Vitamins A, C and E. These vitamins are part of the antioxidants that are used in most cosmetic products. Vitamins A, C and E fight free radicals and maintain the beauty and elasticity of the skin. In addition, they help regenerate the collagen and maintain a firm foundation. Regular consumption of kiwi can delay the signs of aging skin, wrinkles. It also successfully contributes to removing stains caused by the sun. Kiwi fruit is a rich source of dietary fiber, which helps eliminate toxins from the colon and thus detoxify the body. Your skin will look visibly healthier. Helps healing – being a fruit that is rich in vitamin C, regular consumption of kiwi fights inflammation and promotes collagen production. This way, cuts or other wounds will heal much faster. Furthermore, kiwi contains omega-3 fatty acids, compounds which prevent the development of skin diseases. Fights against acne – kiwi fruit pulp contains acids with anti-inflammatory properties that fight bacteria. Other health effects – regular consumption of kiwi fruit lowers the risk of respiratory disease, heart disease, colon cancer; lowers cholesterol levels.

Lavender Oil: Lavender oil relives inflammation in your airways, helps them to widen and allows more air to get through. It can treat cold sores in a few days. Tea made from dried lavender leaves can be useful for headache, upset stomach, depression, insomnia, fungal infections, minor burns and wounds. It can be used to relax in the tub by making a quart of tea to add to bath water or 5-10 drops of lavender oil. Be sure to keep oil out of eyes and not to use for cooking.

Lemon: Lemon is very effective for acne and its related issues. Lemon is a powerful antibacterial agent that discourages the growth of acne-causing bacteria on the skin leaving it fresh and clean. Lemon extracts also act as a natural bleach to lighten the appearance of scars associated with acne giving your skin an even tone. The acid content in lemon helps flush out the toxins accumulations in the pores and helps keep the skin looking fresh. You can either soak a cotton ball in a mixture of lemon juice and water, and clean your skin using it, or take a nice steam that has a few drops of lemon juice in the steam water. It is believed that people suffering from asthma have low levels of Vitamin C and taking lemon may help. Lemons are a rich natural source of Vitamin C, which may also help reduce asthma symptoms. Lemon is also believed to contain some antioxidants that help calm down the inflammation of the internal lining of the respiratory tract, relieving the symptoms associated with asthma. Lemon can be used in any food or drink.

Lemon Balm: Lemon balm is from the mint family and can be used to treat anxiety issues and other stress related problems. It has been used for years to treat insomnia, nausea, headaches, heart problems, indigestion, and as a natural stress reliever. You can find ointments made with lemon balm to help treat insect bites and to clean open sores and cuts. The best way to use lemon balm is to make a tea with the herb and drink it daily to take advantage of its healing properties. You can use lemon balm in its essential oil form and use it as aromatherapy for relieving anxiety, tension, stress, depression, and emotional problems.

Licorice Powder: Licorice Root Extract is from the licorice plants and contains glycyrrhizin, which is a very sweet syrup or powder known to have medicinal properties. It is obtained by pounding the root of the plant, boiling it in water, then evaporating the liquid. The powder is especially helpful in treating eczema and acne. When made into a tea, it is good for digestive or respiratory problems. It is not recommended to have more than 8 ounces of tea in day. Too much licorice can lead to high blood pressure and irregular heartbeat. People with high blood pressure or who are pregnant should avoid it.

Manuka Honey: Mānuka honey is a monofloral honey produced from the nectar of the mānuka tree. Manuka honey treats the flu and is used as a natural ointment for wounds. It is a germ fighter in an age of resistance to conventional antibiotics. It has been known to treat other conditions such as acne and sinus issues.

Nettle Leaf: Nettle leaf has a soothing effect on your joints and naturally relieves pain. It is a potent antihistamine (a substance that blocks the action of histamine, which is a chemical that gets released during allergic reactions and causes many of their unpleasant symptoms). It is best used in a tea.

Olive Oil (Extra Virgin): Extra Virgin Olive Oil is rich in monosaturated fats that are good for protection from type 2 diabetes, helps reduce high blood pressure, protects against red blood cell damage, helps keep bones healthy guarding against osteoporosis, is full of antioxidants for skin health, helps in digestion and controlling weight, prevents protein from damaging cells of major organs, helps keep ears clear of wax and from earaches, lowers the risk of cancers and depression, and can keep your hair from being frizzy. Another big plus is the anti-inflammatory properties that is a natural pain reliever.

Oatmeal/Colloidal Oatmeal: Colloidal oatmeal is simply oatmeal that has been finely ground. The popular use for colloidal oatmeal is in the bath. You can grind 2 cups of oatmeal in a coffee grinder and add it to his bath water. It has properties that comfort itching, so it is a good choice for relieving the pains of eczema and psoriasis. Soak in the bath for ten to fifteen minutes. When you are ready to get out of the bath, be careful as the bathtub will be slick. When drying, don't rub but pat yourself dry with a clean towel. This treatment can be taken up to three times daily to help ease the dry, itchy skin.

Onion: Onions are in the same family as garlic and are an effective natural remedy that help relieve bronchitis. It is believed that the expectorant effect of onions loosens the mucus and phlegm that causes chest congestion and makes breathing easier. Onions are an effective treatment against asthma as they possess wonderful anti-inflammatory properties that reduce the constriction of the airway. The sulfur content in the onions also helps reduce inflammation of the lungs. Eating raw onions is a remedy to make breathing easier for asthma patients and it can prevent build-up of mucus.

Oregano Oil: Oregano oil comes from the leaves and flowers of the oregano plant, which is a perennial herb and member of the mint family. It clears your sinuses and boosts your immune system to help speed up recovery from a sinus infection and remove thrush from the mouth. It can treat foot or nail fungus, yeast and urinary tract infections as well as treat sore throat, cold sores, dandruff and other skin problems.

Papaya: The juice of raw papaya is effective for many skin ailments like corns, warts, pimples and swellings. Also, for diseases like ringworm, applying a paste of ground papaya seeds will help it heal. The unripe papaya can help treat menstrual irregularities and stimulate proper menstrual flow. It can be used as an excellent face mask to hydrate the skin. It has enzymes that are in many cosmetic, skin and hair care products.

Passionflower: Passionflower is a herb found to be effective against many symptoms associated with fibromyalgia, particularly anxiety, stress, tension and insomnia. It can be used to ease hot flashes, withdrawal symptoms and pain.

Peppermint: Peppermint is an effective decongestant that can clear nasal passages and relieve any inflammation from allergies. Peppermint increases saliva production and protects against dry mouth.

Pineapple: Pineapples contain bromelain, an enzyme that can be a meat tenderizer and medicine. Most of the bromelain content of a pineapple can be found in its stem. Bromelain reduces inflammation by lessening the spread of metabolites that promote inflammation. It also relieves and repairs the inflammation of sore muscles after exercising through its high potassium levels and helps in preventing allergies and cancer.

Potato: Potatoes are good sources of potassium, which helps lower and stabilize blood pressure. Potassium is highest in and near the skin and that's why it is good to eat skin. They also contain calcium, iron, Vitamin A, B and C, and phosphorus. They are filling and good as diet food as long as the butter, cheese and sour cream is kept to a minimum amount; however, these are great to be used for someone trying to gain weight. The pulp from crushed raw potatoes mixed with honey, can work well in skin and face packs. It helps cure pimples and spots on the skin. Apply to burns for quick relief and faster healing.

Red Clover: The extracts of red clover are known for their impressive anti-inflammatory and anti-bacterial properties, which is why, it is often used to deal with tooth infections and toothache. It has also been found that the extracts of this herb could be used to provide energy and boost the immune system. Some studies have also found red clover to be rich in B and C vitamins.

Rosemary: Rosemary moisturizes the mouth and stops it from drying out. Inhaling rosemary oil uplifts the mood and works as one of the best rosemary home remedies to remove mental fatigue and relieve headache as it stimulates blood flow. Rosemary tea reduces depression, fights stress, calms anxiety and boosts memory.

Salmon: Salmon is an excellent source of Omega 3 and is a fatty fish that is high in polyunsaturated fats. It is an excellent source of EPA and DHA Omega 3 fatty acids which are already in active form. Omega 3 acids from wild salmon effectively reduce inflammation by increasing the production of adiponectin, a type of hormone that increases muscle carbohydrate use for energy, metabolism boost and fat burning. Salmon is also a good source of Vitamin B2 which is good for the heart, phosphorous that is great for energy production and protein for muscle building.

Spinach: Spinach contains carotenoids, vitamins C, vitamin E and vitamin K which are all known and common components that battle the cytokines that promote inflammation in the body. One study found that one form of Vitamin E known as alpha-tocopherol lessened the inflammation in patients with coronary artery disease. Vitamin E also reverses the levels of adipokine compounds released by belly fats that are inflammatory. Spinach is high in niacin, zinc, folate, calcium and magnesium and best eaten raw such as in salads or sandwiches.

St. John's Wort Oil: It is an oil infusion of the flowers of St. John's Wort flowering plant which is popular worldwide. St. John's Wort oil is essential oil derived from the plant or a preparation where the wilted flowers are soaked in oil and the volatile components are extracted. This oil is used as a massage oil, but it can also be in other creams, salves, moisturizers, and natural remedies to improve their efficacy. It can be used for insect bites, treating burns, healing wounds, reducing muscle pain and inflammation. It can also be used for boosting immune system, treating sunburn, treating sciatica and fibromyalgia. It should not be consumed internally, as it can have bad side effects.

Thyme: Thyme is a popular herb and is used to flavor many food preparations. The extracts of this herb are believed to be effective in helping the body get rid of mucus, and may help strengthen the lungs, preventing the spread of infection. A fourth of a teaspoon of thyme taken with honey, can help curb congestion.

Tomatoes: Tomatoes are excellent sources of lycopene, which is a bright red carotene and carotenoid pigment found in tomato skin. Lycopene inhibits HMGB-1, or a protein that is secreted by activated cells that surround and digest cellular debris and pathogens to prevent the production of inflammation. Lycopene is also an anti-cancer and helps depression.

Turmeric: This spice is a member of the ginger root family and is known for its anti-inflammatory effects. In fact, in India, it is widely used for arthritis and joint pain relief. A main compound of turmeric, curcumin, has been shown in at least 30 different studies to have anti-tumor/anticancer and antioxidant effects. This spice has also been shown to be a wonderful detoxing agent for the liver. Curcumin gives Turmeric its bright, yellow-orange color and its antioxidant and anti-inflammatory properties. Several studies have proven that curcumin actively prevents the triggering inflammatory pathways by stopping the production of two pro-inflammatory enzymes, COX-2 and 5-LOX. Curcumin also prevents cognitive decline, heart diseases and liver damage. Known for its impressive anti-inflammatory properties, turmeric is an effective remedy against cough associated with bronchitis. Adding a small spoon of turmeric powder to a glass of milk before drinking it can help expel the mucus that may have built up in the respiratory tract. When added to foods, it can help reduce pain associated with fibromyalgia.

Valerian: Valerian is one of the best herbal remedies used to deal with fibromyalgia as it relieves muscle tension and weakness and induces sleep. Many other symptoms associated with fibromyalgia including brain fog, concentration problems and decreased focus can be dealt with by taking the extracts of valerian root as a remedy.

Wheatgrass Juice: Wheatgrass is the freshly sprouted first leaves of the common wheat plant. The leaves are processed to be sold as a dietary supplement or as a powder or juice often used in smoothies. It contains all minerals known to man, and vitamins A, B-complex, C, E, l and K. It is effective in healing because it rich in protein containing 17 amino acids. Wheatgrass aids the body in getting rid of impurities, helps the digestive system and can boost metabolism and aid in weight loss.

Witch Hazel: Witch hazel is extracted from the leaves and bark of the North American shrub *Hamamelis virginiana*. It contains powerful tannins, which have astringent and antioxidant properties. The Native Americans used it thousands of years ago as a traditional medicine to treat all kinds of inflammation and tumors. It has become a part of many commercial cosmetics and medical products such as acne products, anti-aging creams, shaving creams, and shampoos. It has properties that are highly active free radical scavengers and help treat and prevent skin cancer and melanoma. It soothes inflammation, redness, and pain due to sunburns, rashes, atopic dermatitis, boils, and blisters. Evidence shows that regular application of witch hazel can help prevent stretch marks and keep the skin moisturized.

White willow bark (the original aspirin): Before there was aspirin there was white willow bark. The Greek physician Hippocrates wrote about it all the way back in 5th century BC. It wasn't until about 1829, that white willow was found to be so effective because it contains an active ingredient called salicin. Salicin is converted in the body into salicylic acid, which is similar to acetyl salicylic acid, the active ingredient in aspirin. Because the naturally occurring salicin is converted after it passed through the stomach, it resulted in less irritation/side effects. While it can be taken in a capsule form, taking it in a tea is very effective.

Chapter 10: Index

9 781790 492770